Surrender to

Alessandra de Lyte

About this Book

In *Ian's Surrender* we learn of a boy born to inherit vast riches who falls into the hands of his scheming step-mother and her daughter with a plot to persuade him to surrender his manhood to them to become a 'husband-slave'.

In *Steel and Stockings... ...Or Slipping into Skirts*. We read a series of encounters of the sort that lead men down the path of surrender to strong women, for them to be feminised, to serve women and men in every way, to be slaves.

Copyright Notice

Copyright 2012 Academy Incorporated Limited, PO Box 135, Hereford, HR2 7WL, UK. All rights reserved. All characters in this story are fictitious. Any resemblance to real persons, living or dead, is purely coincidental. Published by De Muir Press an imprint of Academy Incorporated Limited, PO Box 135, Hereford, HR2 7WL, UK. No part of this document may be reproduced, stored in a retrieval system, or transmitted in any form or by any means without the prior written permission of the publisher. This document may not be circulated in any form of binding or cover other than that in which it is published without all conditions, including this condition, being imposed on the subsequent purchaser. Stories relate to fantasies of freely consenting adults, and despite what you see in this or other books, videos, etc. keep it safe, sane and consensual!

Table of Contents

Surrender To Slavery ··1
   About this Book ···3
   Copyright Notice ···5
   Table of Contents ···7
Ian's Surrender ···9
   Chapter 1 ··9
   Chapter 2 ···13
   Chapter 3 ···24
   Chapter 4 ···28
Steel and Stockings… ···33
   I ···33
   II ··36
   III ···39
   IV ···42
   V ··44
   VI ···48
   VII ··51
   VIII ···54
   IX ···57
   X ··60
   XI ···63
   XII ··65
   XIII ···68
   XV ··72
   XVI ···75
   XVII ··78
   XVIII ···80
Academy Incorporated ··83

Ian's Surrender

Chapter 1

"Ah" said Lady Constance, "here are the young people."

Her daughter Catherine led the way with charm and grace.

"This is Catherine, whom you've heard so much about."

"My darling" said Eveline, embracing her friend's daughter, "you are most delightful."

"Thank you" said Catherine bashfully.

"How old are you, sweet?"

"Just 17, Lady Eveline."

"17! Ah, in the very bloom and blossom of life." But in fact, Lady Eveline Mountjoy de Hortensia was herself, at 40, exceptionally beautiful and very commanding in appearance.

"And are you at school still?"

"Yes, at Honoraria's."

"In Kent?"

"Yes, Lady Eveline."

Truly Catherine was a picture. For the occasion she wore a most fetchingly simple long Summer dress in white which actually allowed one to see her naked form through its material if the Sun were behind her as one looked. But in the drawing room this was not visible.

The ladies continued to fuss over Catherine and then Lady Constance remarked, "And this young man is Ian, my stepson, Arthur's son."

The three women turned towards the shyly bashful waiting form dressed in shirt, tie and grey flannel trousers and there was silence.

"Catherine, introduce your step-brother" said Lady Constance.

"This is Ian" she said plainly.

"Step forward, boy" said Lady Constance "and shake Lady Eveline's hand."

Very gauche, he tried to introduce himself.

"And are you yet fourteen?" asked Lady Eveline haughtily.

"I'm sixteen."

"Sixteen?!! Can it be true?"

The women laughed slightly.

"Really? Sixteen?"

"He looks less."

"Is he well-behaved?"

"Certainly. His sister is helpful in this."

"Ah." The women exchanged knowing looks.

"So Ian" said Lady Eveline, "what are you planning to become?"

"I would like to be a soldier, madam."

"A soldier?"

"Like my father."

The women laughed and Ian blushed.

"But darling, your hair is too long for a soldier's" said Lady Eveline.

"Mama will not let it be cut."

"Quite right for a boy your age."

Catherine smirked.

"Well, young men are adapted for life in different ways" said Lady Constance, "we shall see."

The children presently left the grown-ups, who then resumed their conversation.

* * * * *

"Well Eveline? What do you think?"

"Certainly! Quite possible! You know, young Catherine is the key."

"I thought you would say that!"

"Hasn't she developed wonderfully!"

Lady Constance smiled.

"So elegant! Quite unusual in today's crude and vulgar world."

There was a long pause.

Both women sipped tea.

"I would proceed at once Constance."

"You think so?"

"I do."

Again they sipped tea and nibbled 'Nice' biscuits.

"How long is it since Arthur's death?"

"Six months now" said Constance.

"Six months!"

"And he inherits at eighteen!"

"All that oil revenue!"

"Quite."

"Naturally" said Eveline, "our plans for the boy are quite unconnected to any wealth he may inherit."

"Absolutely."

"In any case, it's only a matter of….. what? two hundred million?"

Both women laughed, then looked cold and grim.

"Quite."

Eveline continued. "To me he looks malleable and ductile, like a piece of copper waiting to be bent."

They again laughed. Neither was trained in basic science; but both had experience of 'bent coppers' as it were. In the one case Superintendent Fitzroy McAllan of the Metropolitan Police and, in the other, Charlie Toogood, chief of the anti-terrorist police of the Nudgeley district of Kennelworth.

"Well," said Eveline, "my disposals are at your service."

This was an old joke between the ladies, a throwback to their days at 'Dean Row', the exclusive girls' boarding school where they spent many a happy hour on the cricket field or riding.

"It's a question of power, Eveline."

"Quite, Connie."

"So you think a measured step by step approach?"

"Yes darling. Begin at once. The whole thing must be surreptitious and slight at first. Catherine will certainly agree to help."

"Then slowly….."

"Slowly draw him deeper in; and if you feel him slipping, then….."

"Shock and awe!"

They laughed.

12

Chapter 2

Lord Arthur had died unexpectedly at 68, supervising British Government Aid to the Middle East. It had all been a great surprise. He had gone purely on humanitarian enterprises – nothing to do with oil revenues and supplies, naturally. The British influence has nothing of self-interest, only fair play and freedom.

Ian admired his military father. When he had been conceived, General Sir Arthur Fotheringay had been chief of the cadet training school at Seafirth and about to receive his peerage. It was during the great campaign (which it turned out he helped finance) to elect our present government. Sir Arthur (as he then was) was still with Lady Muriel and their divorce was a great shock to her. Less so to Sir Arthur, for Muriel was his fourth wife. Constance, with her own baby daughter, became his fifth – and he had beaten his record by staying with her for sixteen years, until his untimely death last year.

Catherine (who had always felt very dependent on her mother and was well aware that her younger step-brother stood to inherit everything) began to sense, like her mother, that time was short. In fact just two years or so, until Ian turned eighteen.

It was all quite clear from the will. Until he was eighteen, Lady Constance was in complete charge of the estate and Ian's upbringing. So by then his outlook on life must be completely in the hands of his step-mother and step-sister.

* * * * *

Lady Constance and her daughter were shopping in Firthwood, the expensive shopping mall.

"Catherine, there is a lot to be said (when one is an attractively beautiful teenager) for displaying one's charms in a subtle way."

They were admiring a skirt in the window of Gondard's, an extremely expensive clothing store.

Catherine smiled. It certainly was very short.

"But mother," she said, "I meet few people. Why should I want to attract the attention of men?"

"Darling, you will not always be at school. Soon you will spread your wings, go to university and it is as well to know how your looks will be received."

Catherine looked at her mother. "To be in control both of your looks and of their reception."

"But mother, isn't a skirt like this – I mean the colour, such a red; the shape and form, calling for attention from uncontrolled eyes?"

"Quite" said her mother.

"But at present I see only my step-brother. He would then become the only one affected by my appearance."

Lady Constance smiled.

"Suppose" said Catherine, gently stroking her shapely and powerful looking jeans – which gave her an almost sporty look, "suppose I were to confront Ian in such a skirt. Suppose he were to become….. to become….. interested, in a way that would be inappropriate for a step-brother?"

"Then he would have to learn control" said his step-mother.

"Oh" said Catherine pensively. A smile of pleasure crossed her expression.

"Yes, he would have to learn control. This duty was laid on me by his father – self-control."

"But wouldn't I be inflaming his lack of control?"

"What better way is there for him to learn true control? After all, those hoping to be fire engine operatives have to ignite fires in order to learn how to counter fire."

They went in; tried the skirt and felt satisfied. At £75 it was reasonably priced. In the Philippines, in our 'economic colonies', women had laboured sewing in dingy rooms so that the new aristocracy may appear beautiful.

"Tonight we are having a little supper party – casual. I want to see you light some fires, darling" said Lady Constance.

* * * * *

True enough. All eyes followed Catherine in her skirt. The red flashed and sparkled; its flimsy flared hem drawing all male eyes to her shapely legs, black very expensive stockings and high heels.

Wickedly, she smiled demurely, slanting her eyes with innocent dissimulation. But she was not unaware of her step-brother. Normally remote from him, she entered sweetly and teasingly into a mock-confederacy of conversation with him as if he were her best friend.

Ian was quite unable to orientate himself towards her new charming self. (In truth, their time under the same roof was often limited as both attended separate boarding schools.) But she had been a rather aloof figure – until now!

Even the kiss, playful and jocular, was unexpected. It lasted a shade too long to be a joke and created an effect that Ian, at sixteen, could not quantify or control. It prevented him sleeping that night and told him of that red skirt's effect on his consciousness.

Catherine enjoyed experiments (being very adroit at science.) Her experiments now became, under her mother's guidance, directed towards affecting her step-brother strongly and indelibly.

He became like wax. On him she imprinted images of herself in various guises and in various costumes.

Unbeknown to him he had become a 'tabula rasa' or 'table-shaped razor' – otherwise called a blank slate, or putty – on which she squeezed effects of her actions indelibly.

Light, apparently innocent touches; games of Ping-Pong for which she wore a short, pleated skirt; jeans with sexy turn-ups; tight tops; and a very subtle increase in make-up. On a very hot day she wore a bikini and spent time in the swimming pool with her step-brother.

Slowly he was inculcated into the web of her attraction. He felt her 'magnetic field' all around him. He was beginning to find his thoughts filled with Catherine.

And then her friend Rachel came for a day.

* * * * *

Rachel was 20, in her last year at university, and surprisingly athletic; six feet tall and broad shouldered, the sort of girl who climbs mountains and scuba dives.

It was strange how out of things Ian suddenly felt as Rachel and Catherine walked arm in arm about the grounds. But the three of them went together for a walk to Grange Hill, which was pleasant enough. They sat at the top and surveyed the countryside below.

"Let's take a picture," said Rachel. "Damn" she went on, "I've left the camera in my bag."

"Where?" said Catherine.

"At that tree where I stopped for a pee."

"Oh, darling Ian," said Catherine, "please run and get it for us."

Only too anxious to please, Ian slipped off. As he returned, he saw them lying next to each other. Was it true? Was Rachel's hand on his step-sister's jeans? He could not quite see clearly. They moved as he approached.

"Oh thank you, darling" said Catherine.

That evening, Catherine drove Rachel back to London.

"Well" said the athletic girl before she left, "nice to meet you, young Ian. See you again."

Ian had settled down to watch TV when his mobile phone went.

"Darling" said Catherine's voice. "Could you check in my bedroom. Has Rachel left a bag there?"

He went upstairs. There was a denim bag lying on the bed.

"Yes" he answered.

"OK. So long as it's safe. I'll get it when I come home – I'll be late."

* * * * *

Alone, he examined the bag. Why did he? It was quite ordinary. There was nothing special; a spare purse, a mirror and a magazine.

Slowly he drew it out.

It was glossy.

* * * * *

Could it be? On the front were two smiling women, hand in hand.

Ian's hand began to shake. 'New Women' was the title. He opened the magazine. 'How Tessa and I became woman and wife.' Good Lord!

He turned several pages, until he came to a section entitled 'Men.' Inside there was a story. Unwillingly, he found himself reading.

'It is important for a New Woman World that men are taught how to submit to us and a good way is to teach them how to submit to each other.

'That's how I got my brother broken in. I introduced him to the rugger captain of our school. My brother's sixteen and sweet. Tim, the rugger captain, loves breaking boys' resistance at my command. So I invited Tim to dinner and sat him next to my kid brother. Tim kissed him on the ear and ran his big hands over my brother's legs. While I watched, he pulled off his trousers and began kneading him.

'He pushed my brother to his knees and made him suck. Then he oiled his bottom and bent him over a chair.

'"Come on sweetie" he said and then stuffed his big cock into my brother.

'I stroked his face gently. "Come on Tim" I teased, "make him scream with joy."

'When it was over and my brother's bottom was full of sticky ooze I made him pull up his pants and trousers and sit in the wetness while I teased and mocked him.'

The article was signed 'Circe.'

. .   .   .   .   .

Next to it, in the same section, was an article by 'John' about how his step-mother had threatened to throw him out unless he agreed to become a 'whore-fag-slut-pussy boy' for her men friends.

He described how he had met 'Jack', the 26 stone beer pot from the 'Hound and Rabbit' and lost his virginity to the gentleman.

Once he had got the taste for it, he had gravitated to 'Matthew', a black guy with the biggest cock in the world (or so he claimed) – fully 1 foot 2 inches long in the dark; i.e. 15 inches!! (?)

John was a mathematics student in 'Quantum variable space functional algorithms' at the time. This cock he described sucking slowly and gently, going into details approximately as one describes volcanic action; i.e. rumbling and eventual eruption etc – lava etc etc. etc. (I need not go into details.)

Then he described how Matthew himself described *his* experience; as one of 'digging deep', as it were.

* * * * *

Naturally, this literary content deeply affected young Ian. He found the images very disturbingly arousing; they, as it were, 'stuck' in his brain as if glued there by psychological intent. He had no idea that this accidental discovery of illicit literature was a well-planned exercise by cunning minds using step-sisterly deviousness.

When Catherine returned next day she asked for the missing bag. "It's Rachel's, you know" she said.

He handed it over to his step-sister.

"I'm seeing Rachel tomorrow. I'll give it to her."

Even without the literary stimulus, Ian found himself re-playing the erotic content. Images flashed through his mind of smiling women hand in hand, watching him embrace and kiss a rugger player type's swelling something or other and gently lick and suck etc.

Self-satisfied, Catherine returned the magazine and duly 'discovered', along with Rachel, that it had been read by unauthorised eyes. Oh horror! How disgraceful! To read one's private material! They laughed.

"I should tell your mother!" said Rachel. "Your wicked step-brother reads your friends' private stuff. *How deplorable!*" They laughed again.

* * * * *

Some days later, Catherine and her mother seemed engrossed in discussion. Young Ian was vaguely aware of something. Shortly after lunch, his step-mother called him as he sat reading in the large garden.

"What are you reading, Ian?" she asked.

"Er nothing" he replied.

"Show me" she said imperiously.

He showed her 'Ships of the Desert' – a book about traders in olden times carrying slaves for sale in exotic lands of the East.

"What curious reading matter" said his step-mother. "Do you have unusual tastes?"

"No Mama" he flushed.

His step-mother smiled regally and led him to her drawing room where Catherine stood, looking happy. She smiled in her cut-off jeans and tank top – they did not smile back. She looked self-satisfied. "Sit" said Lady Constance and Ian obeyed.

Lady Constance was what one must call severely beautiful. Her trousers had that black creased purposefulness which in a woman can seem so much more intimidating because one tends to associate women with something loving and kind.

Lady Constance was a genius with a certain kind of intimidation and needling, undermining questioning. "Ian" she began.

"Yes Mama." (Mama is an outdated form of address, but Lady Constance liked it. She demanded it of her step-son.)

"You enjoy reading?"

He flushed. "Yes Mama."

"Indeed. You like to read" she said, almost to herself. "And what is your favourite reading matter?"

He became uncomfortable.

"Stories, Westerns, key stage four revision papers? What?"

"Er – not exactly."

"Not exactly what?"

"I don't know, Mama."

"I see. And is your reading matter always your own?"

"Yes, Mama."

"Oh." There was a pause. "Then how does it come about that I have a complaint from someone that you have been reading their private material?"

He went very pale.

"Actually?" she said strangely, "perhaps you can explain" she went on. There was a long pause.

"I….." he croaked like a goldfish.

Lady Constance stood up; black in sharp trousers and belt; severe in a tight purple expensive top of t-shirt cut and ankle black boots with pointed high heels. The terrible evidence lay on the table where she had quietly placed it.

"So you like reading, Ian." Silence. "So first, you enjoy prying into your step-sister's friend's private life and second, you read things very evocative of your inner life of desire which greatly shocks and appals me."

He felt sick.

Catherine smiled.

"Your sister's friend is a respectable and highly professional person who one day may reach high in our society with the stern qualities of a tank commander even and you show her respect by stealing her magazine; privately abusing her trust and imbibing this unimaginative filth and vileness. You are in fact in danger of complete corruption and decadent inner collapse and failure, as it were."

Something seemed inconsistent, but before he could speak his step-sister emphasised the point.

"Betrayal" she said to herself, but audibly.

"Naturally; my duty as a step-mother to your father's memory will involve correction and extirpation of your vileness."

"But….." at last Ian broke out." "This is not fair….."

"I must tell you that the police are involved in the question of theft. Luckily for you, a friend of mine is a chief inspector and I may be able to avoid a prosecution – should I deem it wise to avoid one! Or we may let the law take its course."

Ian slumped in his chair, head in hands.

* * * * *

The first of a long series of interrogations and questioning had come to an end. Disgrace can very often be conveyed by silence more effectively than by words.

As the following days revolved, in their wonted revolutionary manner (as Shakespeare, the beard from Stratford in East London says) more was done to the hapless Ian by sending him to a kind of 'Coventry of meaning', then by accusatory expostulations and finally by subtle, needling interrogations.

Lady Constance, with her active past and work for the secret services in Baghdad, supporting the reconstruction of that country by coalition aeroplanes, was an expert at psychological manipulation, inducing by clever pressure what are called 'cracks' in the façade of defence inculcated by traditional educational procedures.

Then it 'became known', by quietly allowing the news to be leaked, that Lady Constance's 'friends' and ex-colleagues General Battenberg and his wife, Commander Phoebe Clay, deputy head of the Metropolitan Police anti-terrorism squad, were coming to dinner.

Naturally, mandatory attendance, which prophetically we might call 'a whip', was served on Catherine and Ian. At the dinner, Ian was treated with the sort of amused charm which those in power enjoy displaying to their victims.

"How delightful you look, darling Catherine" said Commander Phoebe Clay, resplendent in a black trouser suit and severe spectacles. Experience in interrogation radiated from the 55 year old like spiked points.

"My," said General Battenberg, who at 60 looked as grand as the Albert Memorial in his uniform, "I am sure you turn heads, what?"

Catherine smiled.

After several more profuse compliments, Lady Constance said "This is Ian."

"Oh" said Commander Phoebe flatly.

"Quite" said her husband and a cold silence followed.

* * * * *

"Yes" said Commander Phoebe, "sexual life is to be subject to far more stringent control and monitoring than before, now that freedom is spreading."

The General smiled to himself and eyed first Catherine then Ian very obliquely, as if titillated by a thought.

"Darling Phoebe, then let me confess" said Lady Constance.

"Confess?"

"Yes confess. I am deeply concerned over this young man."

"Ian?" she said in mock surprise.

"Yes, Ian."

"But why?"

And then she explained and recounted the whole sorry saga of his misdemeanours.

"Gad!" said the listening General. He stood up in horror. *"Gad!"*

"Calm yourself" said his wife authoritatively and he sat down at once. "Well" said Commander Phoebe Clay (who as one realises retained her maiden name) "well, well" she repeated (twice.)

"Quite" said the General (again.)

Catherine grinned expectantly.

"Darling" said the Commander, "this must be nipped."

"Nipped?"

"In the bud."

"Yes."

"Quickly and severely."

"Ah."

"Sharply."

"But *how*, Phoebe?"

"How?"

"Yes, how?"

"Darling, *punish.*"

"Punish?"

"Punish. Old fashioned, but true."

"Yes?"

"Disgrace!"

"Oh!"

Commander Phoebe continued, "Quickly and maybe Catherine's friend er….."

"Rachel."

"…..Rachel will accept this in lieu of prosecution."

"Prosecution?"

"Do you want Ian on a new order?"

"Order."

"Yes. The government are introducing new 'Nesbos'.

"Nesbos?"

"Yes. No extra-curricular sexual barring orders."

"Good God!"

"Since they are high profile and new, Ian would be sent at once to Nesbo Camp and no doubt journalists would….."

"No!" shrieked Lady Constance.

"Then act quickly."

Ian tried to leave, but his step-mother glared at him and he re-examined his plate of fish.

"Sit where you are, young man" said his step-mother.

"Flogging" said the General. "I've got a whip at home. Used it on my batman when he spilled my brandy."

"No. More subtle I think" said Commander Phoebe Clay.

"Let's discuss it in the lounge" said Lady Constance.

She turned to the 'children'. "You can sit in the drawing room and wait quietly."

"Yes Mama" they said humbly.

* * * * *

Catherine, stunning in a deep blue evening dress, sat opposite her glum step-brother in his black suit.

"Well, Ian" she said.

He looked at the floor.

"I would never have guessed. *You*. Ian. Such a dirty-minded, disgusting….."

He flushed red.

"How do you justify yourself?"

"But….. the magazine….." he stammered. "I mean" he went on, "Rachel….. gay."

"You disgusting pervert!" said his step-sister.

"But….."

She stood up, radiant in her blue dress, eyes sparkling with fiery anger. "Pervert!"

* * * * *

Lady Constance and her friend, Phoebe Clay, derisively planned a re-educating and humiliation of their young victim.

"Do you think that's how to begin then?" said Lady Constance at last.

"Definitely. Extreme chastity is of great importance. There is a continual emphasis on something. On its denial. On the inability to feel. A continual frustration. One is severely punished. When it has done its job, say for two weeks, then something arousing."

Lady Constance smiled.

* * * * *

The little group assembled.

"Sit down, Ian" said his step-mother. "Commander Clay would like to speak to you."

Commander Clay assumed her most authoritative posture. "Well, young man" she said; "well."

Ian flinched and trembled.

"You see, your step-mother has told me all about this er..... incident; as you know. Do you?"

"Yes."

"'Yes, Commander Clay'" snapped his step-mother.

"Yes, Commander Clay."

"Good boy. Well, this is how it stands. The government has, as you know, instituted an action plan for personal developmental improvement. Did you know that?"

"No, Commander."

"'No, *Madam* Commander'" said his step-mother.

"No, Madam Commander."

"Good boy. Well, this is in fact the cause. Thanks to an on-line audit survey modular deposition, it has been decided to introduce a pilot."

There was a strange silence. "A pilot" she repeated. "This is the case. You are being given the chance to take part in the pilot."

Ian pictured a large airman.

"The pilot will be a chance for you to avoid prosecution, if Rachel will agree. She may. Or she may insist on prosecution."

"Oh" said Ian.

"If she prosecutes, then you may escape with six months at a new government democratic boot camp, where you will receive anti-depressant injections of 'xylohexylp-chloruptazine methanologiate' on an hourly basis.

"Oh."

"Have you heard of it?"

"No, Madam Commander."

"Well, it has awkward side effects. But it regularises behaviour very effectively. However, the disgrace for your step-mother and your father's memory….."

"Oh, Madam Commander."

"So, we can ask Rachel if she will sign a form to enlist you in the pilot programme of behaviour control?"

"Thank you, Madam Commander."

"And you will then be part of research for new auditing of the population and improvement programmes."

"Thank you."

"Darling Catherine, let's ask Rachel right now. Could you e-mail her at once and ask her to log on" said her step-mother.

Catherine looked surprised.

Thanks to Phoebe Clay's superior technical knowledge, a mobile phone was used and a contract was signed with a 'logged on' Rachel enlisting Ian in a pilot that very evening.

"Really, you should be very grateful" said Phoebe Clay; "you are to be trained, made useful, made into what society wants. Your own sinful and disgraceful nature will be 'civilised' and made productive."

The matter was settled. Sent to his room, Ian, having proved he was unable to cope with polite society, lay in bed and trembled with fear at the new turn of events, all caused by his wicked desire.

Meanwhile Catherine, in her beautiful evening dress, was informed of the oncoming punishment and modification.

Involuntarily, she laughed. Her piercing note reached Ian, tossing this way and that in his bedroom. But it added to his fear. Catherine was now party to what would happen to him.

What would it be?

Chapter 3

The letter arrived by formal courier. By that is meant, someone from Special Branch. It gave a clinic address in Harley Street, London.

Lady Constance, Catherine and Ian were driven by Butler, the chauffeur, through busy London streets.

Catherine, in black boots and sturdy jeans (at £150) in black denim with gold fringes and a tight black t-shirt from 'Lauren' in the West End and her mother in a long skirt and jacket from 'Estelle Murat' in her new 'Guillotine' range in deep red, got out of the car and ushered Ian, in his flannel trousers and white shirt into the waiting building. (This may cause surprise. Not everyone knows that buildings wait, but it is true. But wait for what?)

Butler settled himself in the car and looked at the Daily Mirror and Sun, beginning on page 2 at 'Philosophical Reflections' and moving on to 'World Problems in Catholic Thought' on page 4, leaving out the icons displayed on page 3 of various quintessentially displayed 'as it weres'.

The trio sat in the waiting room. Expensive patients were summoned in and out of mysterious rooms, while one (token) NHS patient adjusted the tent that she and her child were sleeping in during their six week stay. After 17½ minutes, six seconds inside Government Guidelines, they were called in.

Menacingly efficient nurses bristled smirkingly in the treatment room.

Both Catherine and her mother gazed satisfied at the way Ian was subtly and firmly taken into determined feminine hands. Stripped naked and laid on a treatment table, he was suffered to display his offending organ, which he had indulged in his crime.

"So here's the little perverted gay creature," said a doctor efficiently.

Quietly and firmly she took the organ in her hand and subtly began to manipulate it for medical reasons. She watched as expressions of deep pleasure spread over Ian's face. Then she stopped.

"Now," she said to Lady Constance, "there are two ways to proceed. Either we forcibly 'empty the sacks' as it were and then….. Or, we increase the pressure to its maximum so as to allow immediate need and then prevent it."

"What do you think, Catherine?" she asked her daughter.

Ever the cruel one, Catherine gave her answer.

So some teasing manipulation was suddenly followed by a bag of ice. The actual fitting took very little time.

With modern technology, chastity devices can be fitted with 'gadgets' which can be remotely controlled and soon they were in a London restaurant. With Ian adjusting to the strange sensation (or lack of sensation) somewhere intimate.

* * * * *

"Hi" said Jessica.

Catherine led her friend to the party. She loved parties. Her friends were like her, very nubile and stunning. Young girls have a natural flower that makes it unnecessary for much adornment, but any adornment thus becomes extra specially potent in its effect.

Jessica, in a denim mini-skirt and loose top, showed off her lovely slim legs. Veronica, with big powerful hips, swayed slightly in her shorts and tank top; while Anne, tall and stately in a pair of cut off jeans, marched gracefully.

The girls loved these all-girl parties – they cultivated energy levels and potencies. The music was slow and other-worldly, yet very sensual.

Lady Constance breezed in and chatted for a while, then left them to it. "You will keep an eye on Ian?" she said.

"Ian?" said Jessica. "A boy?"

"Well" said Catherine, "Sort of."

"We can't have any boys Cath, you know that."

Catherine called them into a huddle. In the doorway stood the boy himself in a pair of jeans and a green shirt. They turned and looked, their eyes wide.

"Ooh" said Jessica. They ushered him in.

By 8.30 several more girls have arrived and were surprised to find a boy included in their proceedings. Soon he found himself surrounded by ten or twelve skimpily clad gorgeous teenage girls in every conceivable fashion. Each delighted in arousing the helpless young man, whose frustration and need had steadily increased over a long period of chastity.

"Do you mean to say" said Gloria, "that this boy Ian is….." The words died on her breath.

"Yes. Neutered" said Catherine.

"Wow!"

"For how long?" asked Susan.

"Oh let me see….. it must be three months now."

"Three months with no release?"

Catherine smiled.

"Darling" said Rebecca, "I know it's not fair, but could we….. peep?"

Thus it came about that Ian was made to show his obedience by allowing his hands to be held aloft by two strong girls, while others unzipped his jeans and displayed the strange device which deprived him of all sensations.

The girls all touched it one by one like people touch a new puppy, or stroke a kitten.

"You are so brave to let yourself be neutered like this" said Veronica.

They let him pull up his jeans and sit in humiliated impotence.

* * * * *

As the weeks passed, Ian became increasingly docile and obedient. It is remarkable how deprivation makes a man of you! Well, not quite. In Ian's case it *un*made a man of him!

But slowly control passed into the hands of his temptresses; until Lady Eveline came to inspect progress, bringing with her a strange Asian girl of 30, fresh from training (in America) in techniques of 'adjustment to reality' or 'A.T.R.'

Under direction, Ian passively agreed to the wedding. Naturally, he supposed that his chastity belt might be removed and refitted for the occasion of marriage, but this proved a chimera; as you will hear.

Chapter 4

Viola straightened her skirt and checked her lipstick admiringly. What good fortune to look….. well, very attractive. It had been a great trouble to Lorenzo di Medici to look less than a water colour or egg tempera Venus. But Viola, with her blonde ringlets, was no Lorenzo.

She checked her keys, handbag and remote. Then she was ready. Quickly to the loo, then another skirt straightening in the hall mirror; at last, time to go.

She decided to have one last look. She opened the bedroom door. He turned with a despairing look. Perhaps it was a bit cruel – I mean, he was her husband! She walked over to him and smiled down.

"OK, my pet?" She stroked his face gently.

A touch of doubt. The gag was….. well it was a bit….. well….. *rude*. (It was a new kind, devised by 'CKSOC' for their new range – a bit expensive, but very juicy. It had a delicious taste and would 'ooze' a kind of sweet liquid at regular intervals.) But she had been unsure of the shape. I mean, it was obviously shaped like a male organ.

He gazed away from her – ashamed no doubt – and his eyes rested on her white gypsy skirt, recently washed and then on her red flower dress, both hanging in a wardrobe. She was so beautiful it positively hurt.

Gently she looked at his helpless form. "Darling" she said, "when Vulcan found his wife Venus in bed with Mars, do you know what she did? She tied them up in bed together and invited all the gods to look at them and laugh."

She laughed softly. "Well, you can see we've changed the myth a little! Dear Mars, you'll have to lie there alone while Venus hops off on her own!"

Her perfume was all around her, strong. It seeped into him, carrying her beauty. She turned to go and he saw her beautiful bottom outlined through her short tight skirt.

As an afterthought, she turned and checked his cuffs. Not because they ever came apart, but because it was nice to do it. To feel their comfortable expensive luxurious firmness and inevitability. There was no escape from their comfort.

She delighted in tickling him a little. It always aroused him to be tickled. How silly in a boy of 17! But of course the light tickling in the crease of his elbow or under his arms always did it for him. And his 'little boy' would always try to stand up, but then meet its prison! A wicked urge made her look once more at his new high tech chastity device.

"Happy darling?" she said. "I bet you never suspected what I wanted in a husband, did you?" She drew out the remote from her bag and tested it by depressing button 'A'. It did not produce the sound of coins descending. Instead a sharp twinge shot through the air from the remote and deposited itself in his chastity device. Very effective!

"I don't mean to be cruel" she lied. She pressed button 'B' and the coins did not empty themselves on the floor. Instead a stirring occurred in the (as it were) 'behind' region.

"Just testing" she said sweetly. She straightened herself again. "Time to go, my little love husband."

He gazed longingly.

"Are you going to be good? Think what you would like for a treat tonight. I haven't decided yet. Would you like an evening with 'Clara'? Or perhaps 'Stephanie' should come? Or shall I invite Max round?"

All three produced a look of fear.

She laughed. "Well. Off I go, little husband. Just think about the word. You are my *slave*."

The front door clicked and another long silence began.

* * * * *

Was this marriage? To be tied to a bed, hands and feet held by gentle and commanding cuffs and only able to move inches. To be sucking a male genital shaped organ which oozed liquid. To have a chastity device annulling all feeling in one's own organ and a thing in one's bottom which could vibrate under remote direction.

Was this husband-hood? As he asked this question he could hear the laughter of his wife. Beauteous, lovely, gorgeous, pretty Viola – 30, successful company director, now speeding down the government's new clearway to her work in the City.

As a government employee, Viola had exemption from all restrictions and could do as she liked.

She was just parking in the director's area when she reached for the remote, arranged for a five minute burst of medium power and pressed both 'A' and 'B' (to hear the coins rattle.)

She entered the building and was greeted by the computer. That is to say she was recognised by the clip in her hair slide. The doors opened and a voice greeted her. "Good morning, Ms Trentham."

The production of electronic circuitry for use in missile guidance was becoming more and more secret. Viola Trentham passed along rows of offices in government corridors where information was carefully prepared for public consumption explaining the peace-loving nature of the missile guidance systems and the confusing of propaganda sources of lying stupid racist bigoted 'Shites'.

(The Shites are a branch of 'Al-Turda', the well-known fanatical group of terrorists, under their sinister leader, Hosanna Dustbinlid, who lives in a hole in a part of the Asda Supermarket storeroom in Brodesley, East Birmingham, England.)

Viola passed all these corridors of government security until she reached her office, where only high personnel are admitted.

She sat at her desk and logged on her interactive judgement device for a new batch of cases. As it 'booted' she thought about Ian, her 'husband' slave. "Viola" her mother had said, "every successful woman needs a good wife."

Ian, at 17 was in fact her wife, i.e. her slave. Her skivvy, cleaner and toy. Her grovelling, obedient, helpless victim.

From time to time her mother-in-law, Lady Constance, came to inspect her stepson to see how he was proceeding with marriage and often 'spoke to' Xia, Ian's personal trainer in obedience, to ensure that Ian remembered how to make a happy marriage.

Viola wondered what to do on returning home. Would she bring out 'Clara', she wondered? Ian, helpless in his bondage at home, wondered the same thing. Clara bit devilishly. She was black, three feet long and had a bone handle. His wife adored standing over him and lashing Clara into his skin. Usually three lashes would turn him into a helpless grovelling jelly or even blancmange.

Or perhaps it would be nice to bring out 'Stephanie'. Stephanie was the shy submissive girl her husband became when she wanted a doll to play with.

When *she* was a little girl, Viola used to dress a little doll called 'Barry' in little panties, a bra and short skirts and then smack him fiercely.

But Ian was her *real* doll. She might 'Stephanise' him and then invite Max to come round and let him watch while he fucked her furiously (the idiot.) Or even let him fuck her little doll boy, Stephanie. This would be new territory, however.

The computer screen flashed up 'Case 4623911'. The face appeared on the webcam of a scared looking character, probably 25, in Venezuela. Name, Vincenzo de Potatino.

The statement, read out in a monotone began:

"Accused has been found guilty of passing illicit material to government operatives and inciting 'instruction refusal'. This is a category 'A' offence."

There was a pause. Viola looked at the handcuffed prisoner, thought of her husband and felt very, very powerful.

"Punish." What a strong word. She loved the power of remote judgement. Far away, primitive, underdeveloped countries like Venezuela, Antarctica, Botswana, Germany and Brazil all submitted security cases for democratic judgement.

The offending letter appeared. It had scrawled in hopeless writing the ludicrous words 'Think for yourself'. She laughed scornfully. This clap-trap again!

The prisoner stared at the screen. What he saw was a picture of an impassive woman with the phrase 'Justice and Democracy'. What she saw was a wayward example of human terrorism. She was not enjoying this. Naturally, she told herself that punishment of terrorists was a duty. But it was true she did enjoy punishing her wife. After all, that's what wives are for.

The prisoner was staring helplessly at the screen.

She depressed question X23. "So do you appreciate the undemocratic nature of your activities?"

The reply was processed as V431 and came out as "I deserve punishment and beg mercy. I need re-education." What he actually said was "I want freedom to think."

Quietly Viola selected an appropriate punishment. First she pressed 'Guilty'. Then the word 'Severe'. Next, watching her victim's face as she communicated by flashed up words these directives, she spoke.

"You will be punished severely. Your offence is very severe. Everyone is already free to think. Government directives plainly state that free thinking exists."

She watched his anxious face and quietly selected 'Violation'. This reminded her of something. She decided to watch when the punishment would be meted out, perhaps tomorrow.

Having pressed the key, various pictures came up of 'rapist' operatives – large men with gigantic 'things' which were kept for the purpose of punishment of recalcitrants.

She selected 'Abdul', a huge Turkish bear with a 17 inch weapon, 4 inches thick as the crow flies and laughed cruelly to herself.

The punishment was displayed to the prisoner, who begged for mercy. But the computer translated this as "Thank you. I am guilty."

* * * * *

Viola made a note to watch the video replay of the punishment. It intrigued her to watch the terrified look as prisoners met their fate for 'undemocratic' behaviour. They watched a massive man approach them intent on rape and violation and savoured the moment of submission to democratic impulses.

The day was passing pleasantly. She thought of her husband-wife and sent him a shock of impulses from the remote.

She decided. Tonight he would be her doll. Stephanie. She selected his costume in her mind. Very sexy underwear in pink and a mini-dress. He always looked especially sweet in pink.

She decided to invite Dawn and Ronald to share the evening. Dawn loved sharing the humiliating decoration of her husband, while Ronald watched, amused.

She had taught Ian how to please Ronald. How to *suck*. Gently, she tutored him in the arts of male pleasure. Really it was very humiliating.

Democracy. How we worship it. Everyone is free.

Steel and Stockings...

...Or Slipping into Skirts.

I

She isn't my real sister. She's my step-mum's daughter. Three years older than me. We moved when I was six and then Dad got sent to Iraq and when he came back decided to leave Helen (my step-mum) and she brought me up with her own daughter. That's Kathy.

Being older, she often got to boss me around and I suppose I needed the security. There is security in fear isn't there?

My step-mum started a course. She was only thirty odd after all and so Kathy got a lot of responsibility over me very early and her Mum encouraged it, after all, it kept me quiet and out of the way. Sometimes my aunt Nora would come over and look after us.

But usually Kathy organised me and even sorted out my clothes and things.

"You'll make a terrific mum..." Said Nora to her niece.

I don't suppose any of them realised just how much I was falling under my stepsister's spell. I mean, was it quite natural? She even took me to school and back. Pretty good for a nine-year old, and after a year of this guidance we were getting well set in our ways.

The thing was, Kathy was growing older. Her mother's rein was loose at the best of times, and Kathy was open to the influences that affect little girls these days. She watched young women closely.

At night, Kathy used to read me a story and put me to bed. Can you believe it? I was only seven! She would read me stories like Narnia or Tom's Secret Garden, but I think I was still only seven when she began to change.

Imperceptibly at first, but then more so, she had recently got her place at secondary school and been to visit, and I was aware that she would not be at my school anymore. Would I cope without her?

It must have been towards the end of her last year in primary school when it happened...

It was story-time as usual. She seemed restless as we finished Jack the Tank about an American boy who stole away to Afghanistan to visit his dad, and she started to read me a story she said was written by a friend.

"Who is it?" I asked.

"Oh, someone already at 'Severncoats.' (The secondary school she was due to go to in September.) "She used to be at our school, but now she's fifteen."

I couldn't believe it that Kathy had a friend of fifteen.

"Once upon a time," she began, "there was a boy called Tim. Tim lived with his Mum in a cottage in the country. Tim was a good boy…"

11

"This is your first interrogation." She said.

He stood smartly to interrogation.

"How old are you?"

"Sixteen and a half."

"Sixteen and a half err…"

"What will you call me?"

"Madam."

"Say it…"

"Sixteen and a half, Madam…"

"You can call me 'Sir.'" She said.

He looked surprised.

"Do it."

"Sixteen and a half Sir."

"Now, tell me about when you first knew."

He swayed slightly and remembered.

"I was about ten when my sisters…"

"Sisters?"

"Yes; they're two and four years older. They bought a new collar and lead for the dog. They wanted to try it on me to see if it would fit."

"So they…"

"Yes. It was not very tight. But then my older sister fastened the lead and pulled me to the floor."

"And?"

"I tried to take it off, but my other Sister bound my wrists together with a belt and I was helpless."

"And you…"

"Liked it."

"Liked it."

"Sir." He added.

"We will have to extend that experience."

He looked scared.

"Then what else?" She commanded.

He looked at her jeans. They showed her immense dominance. Her lips were strong and rounded and powerful. His eyes drank denim.

"Then they… When I was about twelve, they began dressing me up."

"How?"

"As a girl."

"They started them?"

"Well, when I was younger they began in little ways."

"Go on."

"When Jessica had a pair of shorts she made me wear them once. Sir. And Sophie made me wear an old dress she'd grown out of. Sir."

"And you liked it?"

"Yes Sir."

"You want to be a girl?"

"Yes Sir."

"To serve."

"Yes Sir."

"Because you are only average. Not that clever. You are born to serve, to wait, to obey, to be ordered to be controlled, to slave like a silly girl, like a bitch on a lead, to be trotted out, and used by all the dogs in town."

"Yes Sir."

III

"This is your second interrogation."

"Yes Sir."

"Do you like the process? It's now two weeks since you signed the agreement. Do you want to proceed?"

"Yes Sir."

"Good. You are recognizing your own nature."

"Yes Sir."

"Shall I be cruel to you?"

"No Sir, please."

She smiled.

"Why not?" She smoothed her severe black skirt over her legs.

"I am frightened."

"You will find I am cruel sometimes, and I will be towards you."

He did not reply.

She went on.

"Cruelty will be good for you. You will crave it. Long for my cruelty, for my devious control, for my ruthless determination to subdue you."

"Yes, Sir."

"To crush your resistance, to wrong-foot you and snap you until at a click of my fingers you will run to me and obey."

"Yes, Sir."

"You will be a certain aspect of girl. Of the feminine, not the part that real women have. Strong, mature, regally beautiful, intelligent and commanding. You will have the part that men lust after, weak, submissive, accepting, demure, helpless and supportive. You will be totally dependant on a strong figure, and I will make you so obedient, but also so alluring, so attractive, simpering, empty headed, so crushed into abject attractiveness, no-one will resist staring at you in lustful urge, to use and enjoy you...

...This will be your slavery, to be a doll for someone else. For a stupid ignorant man, or for a Mistress who will own you, play with you and discard you. How do you like the idea?"

"Very much, Sir."

"Well then, you must get used to cruelty. When your owner dresses you up like a prize flower or bitch in a dog show and shows everyone your total devotion to obedience and people admire your utter submission."

"Yes, Sir."

"Tell me, when did you first notice this in yourself?"

"When I was fourteen… We played football against another school. I was hopeless. I was usually put in as a substitute for the best player who was ill. I let a player on the other side score. Our boys were furious with me after the match. I was roughed up, but on the way home, one boy pitied me as I cried. Then he…"

IV

"So, you're a City Councillor then?" She said.

He nodded. She reckoned he was about fifty-three or fifty-four.

"And director of sixteen companies." He added.

"Imagine!" She said.

"I'm a man of importance."

"Quite so."

She accepted the cash.

"I need to be very discreet." He said.

"Obviously."

She led the way into a plush sitting room with two huge armchairs in black leather, which seemed to embrace you.

"Please sit down Councillor."

He sat.

She pressed a little bell and a door at the other end opened.

The councillor looked at the demure figure, eyes down, approached shepherded by a very attractive blonde figure. The boy, in fetching jeans and black shoes knelt before the Councillor:

"Now. Slowly unzip his trousers."

The boy obeyed. Gently, very slowly, as he had been taught, unzipping the man's front.

"Now, feel inside." She said.

It was already big. Swaying a little. As shown, he began to rub and knead. Feathery touches on the skin, then pulling back the foreskin, he gasped.

He continued. Gentle teasing, kneading. She gave a sign.

Gently, he pressed his mouth towards it, hardly sucking, pursing lips and licking. Then rubbing again. He took it in a little way, licked all around and then withdrew.

The Councillor gasped. Again, he rubbed, and then licked the man's balls. He stroked, rubbed and licked. The man gasped on… 'Gasp! Gasp!'

Again, he pressed it in, sucked and pushed his cheeks. She smiled at her expert teaching. She wanted the Councillor to feel completely enthralled.

Possibly ten or fifteen minutes passed. He continued devotedly sucking, kneading and stroking, following prior instruction and teaching. At last the Councillor groaned. A feeling of power swept over him, but his Mistress at once took this away. She had created everything. She was the at-one-remove power source.

"Oh, bloody fantastic!" Said the Councillor. "Fantastic!"

She led out the slave. She was already reckoning his price would be considerable when further training was complete.

She gave him a diploma in C.S. or B.J.

"So." She said. "Would you like to know how you are doing?"

She was in an elegant red evening dress and matching high-heels.

"Since taking weekly interrogations and tutorials and attending lectures and demonstrations for a period of four weeks." She read. "The candidate has revealed a submissive and obedient nature. There is good promise of a successful outcome. The candidate has elements of slavery naturally in place and others can be developed when obstructive factors have been destroyed." She put down in the notes…

"…So basically," she continued, "you are doing fairly well. I was pleased with your practical. It was your first?"

"Yes, Sir."

"The Councillor is an old fart, but we need him on side and he wants to visit you again, probably tomorrow or Wednesday."

"Yes, Sir."

"You don't like him do you? I know, he smells of smoke even down to his socks."

"Yes, Sir."

She looked at her watch: Six-Thirty-Four.

"What time does your aunt expect you?"

"She doesn't expect me. If I stay out all night, she doesn't notice. I'm free."

"I am going out to an expensive dinner at seven-thirty."

She pondered a little. "Wait there and I'll speak to you in a moment."

"Yes, Sir."

After a few minutes she returned with a young woman in a short skirt, perhaps twenty-five. "This is Estelle," she said.

The young woman was short and stocky with fizzy hair. "Come here and say 'hello.'"

He got up and walked to the two women. As he reached them, she placed a hand on his head and pushed him down.

"Down," she said, "on your knees."

He sank to his knees.

"Now, ask Estelle to take care of you."

"Please, please Estelle, take care of me."

"Will you obey me?" Said Estelle.

"Yes Miss."

"Good."

Estelle carried a little shopping bag. Inside there were, a pair of girls shorts in crimson satin. "Go and put these on and come back to me."

Nervously, he obeyed. They were tight and uncomfortable, but at once he discovered, he began an erection.

He zipped them up, but it was horribly uncomfortable. The two women looked up at him. His legs were long and shapely and hairless. They smiled.

"Comfortable?" Said Estelle.

"Yes." He lied.

"Kneel." She said.

He knelt.

"Eyes closed."

He obeyed.

The collar was somehow reassuring and very familiar.

She came in behind him. He could feel her red dress against his skin. She undid his shirt and pulled it away, replacing it with a kind of vest with straps for shoulders.

He knelt between the two women. Then he felt something on the collar and a little tug. He knew it was a lead. He did not resist. From behind she forced his wrists together and with some kind of sash, tied them.

"Obedience." She said to herself.

"Open your eyes." Said Estelle.

He saw her smiling down at him lead in hand.

She led him to a wall mirror.

"See?" She said.

With a black collar and lead and tied hands he saw himself. On the black T-shirt was written in gold: Slave Bitch.

In her red dress, she came alongside and the mirror reflected the three figures. The women led him by the lead to the door and downstairs. It was dusk.

She picked up her handbag and looked at her watch.

Presently, a car hooted.

"I must go." She said.

The women exchanged glances.

Outside the house was a driveway. She looked in the hall mirror, arranged her hair and added some lipstick. Then turned to him. She rearranged his hair a little, then gently holding his face close, cradled in her arm whispered "Be beautiful for me," and ran the lipstick over his lips carefully. She smiled and sprayed perfume over him.

"I must go."

But Estelle pulled the lead and all three went towards the car. It was cool in the driveway. They pulled the garden gate and she climbed in and waved.

She smiled and waved.

Estelle looked at him.

"This way!"

To his horror she started down the street.

He hung back.

She pulled.

He tried to dig his heels in.

She came up to him.

"I can't." He whispered. He stood frozen to the spot.

A middle-aged couple were approaching. As they got level she made sure she did not obstruct the view of his T-shirt.

They tried not to look.

Then she came behind and delivered a fierce smack.

He found himself walking. She pulled.

After a circuit of the residential block where they passed only two or three people, she headed off towards Queen Street. They passed cafés, the supermarket and garage.

She loved it when people stared. Better if they laughed. She led him into a café in Brompton Street.

"In!"

She sat and drank a cola. It was evidently pretty Bohemian. People just smiled at the obedient figure, hands tied, with a collar and lead and a T-shirt announcing 'Slave Bitch.'

She led him back through the city-centre and by now he was inured to the laughs, smiles, nudges and comments.

They got back home.

"Good boy!" She said and patted him.

She kept him on the lead.

She sat and watched television and he lay at her feet.

She let him relieve himself, but he had to undo his shorts. She fastened them, but he was still erect. She teased his erection, made it more uncomfortable and made sure the shorts were tight around it.

"Beddy Byes!" She said.

She pulled him to a kind of storeroom where a mat was laid. She tied the lead fairly tight around a table-leg and told him to lie on the mat under the table.

Then she put the light out and shut the door.

He was then aware of a voice. There was a tape player or something in the room.

A voice began.

"I serve my Mistress. She leads me into her web of slavery. I obey. I am her weak slave. She consumes me in her desire. She controls me. She is my Queen. She makes me do things to men. She makes me love to take men in my mouth. To suck and lick them. She loves to see me serve men and lick them. She adores seeing me fucked hard. Men fuck me. Their dicks enter me throbbing, pushing and vibrating…"

The shorts were by now very uncomfortable.

"She is my controller, she dominates me. I belong to her. I cannot escape. I am a slave. There is no release…"

VI

"Tell me."

"Well… When I was fourteen, just two years ago… She was eighteen I think."

"Who?"

"She was called Marcia."

"And…?"

"She worked as an assistant at school. She was a drama student."

"And…?"

"We were doing a play. She told me I had to play a girl."

"And…?"

"So I did. She was called Anna."

"The student?"

"No. The part."

"And…?"

"So I read the part. The others laughed. I blushed."

"And…?"

"She told them to be quiet. Reassured me. Then we tried it in costume."

"Tell me."

"It was a skirt of hers. Straight. Quite long, white, with a matching jacket. The kids whistled. I felt strange."

She smiled.

"Did you feel naughty?"

"Yes, Sir."

She slowly pulled down his jeans and lightly caressed and teased his bottom.

"Did she do this to you?"

"No, Sir. She would have been in trouble."

"But did you want her to? To run her nails over your bottom, to tease you?"

"Yes, Sir."

"Like this?"

"Oh, yes Sir!"

"To wear her white panties. Her bra."

No answer.

"Well, you shall, darling slave. You will wear panties and bra and a straight white skirt, and jacket and blouse. You will wear stockings and high-heels just like she did."

She pulled on his collar.

"Now lick my boots."

He licked. Images swirled. He saw himself in white panties, bra, stockings, a skirt, make-up; just like her.

"Anna." She said.

Then she pulled him over her knee and spanked furiously.

Then again, teasing caresses, then: Spank! Spank! Spank!

Tiny feathery strokes.

She laughed.

The door opened.

"Get up Anna!"

"Gabriel and Lucy." She introduced. "They are going to make you into Anna. The girl you are on the inside."

He followed submissively.

VII

She wore a black skirt and stockings. Her heels dug the carpet. A pendant hung around her neck, a picture on it of a boy asleep while a woman stood over him.

"Look."

She sat opposite him in a hard backed chair. From behind a figure approached. She nodded. The figure produced a little white pill.

"Eat."

Nervously.

"You look lovely," she said, "pink suits you." The dress was short. The hem caressed the pale tights above the knee. The lips were luscious.

"Gabriel is clever. You look ever so girlish."

The voice seemed to come from the table behind. The clock started to laugh. The sea beneath her heels became a carpet for a minute and…

"Hold her."

It seemed someone was giggling uncontrollably.

"Listen."

"Sex," said a voice urgently, "furious determined sex. Sex, sex, sex!"

The giggling did not stop.

"A man. A man he will take and use. Want, desire, be possessed."

Someone was kneeling.

Laughter.

"Oh, my lovely dress," said a voice.

It went on.

"I am a girl. I feel so fucking sexy. Oh, please fuck me. FUCK ME!"

"Feel my dress. Like pink cream. Oh, fuck. Fill me."

"What do you want, pet?"

"A man. To fuck and fuck me. To spear me. Oh, fuck."

Laughter.

"Please."

"Please what, pet?"

"Oh, please, I need a man. I need… I need… I need."

They laughed.

"You shall have one, pet. A big strong hunky hulk, a giant with a club who will stick it in you."

"Oh, yes, yes, yes!"

Laughter.

The world swirled.

* * * * *

"How do you feel?

"Strange sir."

"Oh!"

She pressed a remote and the play back shone on the screen.

"That's you!" She said. "Look how you lift your dress, pull down your panties and…"

He looked in dumb silence.

"Quite a little slut!"

He pouted his beautifully pink lips and felt something.

VIII

"We understand you very well."

"Yes, Sir."

"Yes. We know you and your needs. Your type."

"Yes, Sir."

"We know your weaknesses."

"Yes, Sir."

She wore an elegantly feminine long white skirt.

"You are to be sold."

"Sold?"

"On trial. Would you like that?"

"I am not sure."

She laughed.

"To a certain Lady Fitzallan. Her daughter is sixteen. Your age. She needs a servant. Someone to punish and play with."

She laughed.

"You start tomorrow. It's in Gloucestershire."

"Yes, Sir."

"Lady Fitzallan is concerned about your lack of control."

"Yes, Sir."

"She does not intend her daughter to be in any way defiled by you."

"No, Sir."

"So you will be fitted."

"Fitted?"

"Yes. Under your skirts."

"Yes, Sir."

Later that day he stood in his short cotton skirt and then she said, "There, how does it feel?"

It was strange, deep underneath his pretty panties.

"It denies all release. You can rub all you like. You will feel nothing."

She laughed.

"Now you must go to have your hair done. I want Penelope to be pleased with you."

"Penelope?"

"Your new young Mistress. Run along!"

He emerged a mass of fluffy curls, a sort of white-icing creation in a long white skirt. The sort of thing young girls wear to look grown up.

She smiled.

"Lady Fitzallan has been told of your more positive properties."
"Yes, Sir."
"This is a test."
"Yes, Sir."
He ran his hands down his long skirt.

IX

Penelope Fitzallan, utterly upper class 'Modern Miss' with a born-to-rule mentality wore a pair of shapely black trousers, stockings, mules and a loose blouse.

Her friend, Anne Springers and she attended Priors, a tertiary college for exclusive ladies.

The taxi dropped them at Fitzallan Hall where Anne was staying the weekend with her friend.

"You must get one, Anne."

"My God Penny, I can't believe it."

"He is completely docile."

"I must see."

She had told her best friend that her mother had given her…

"We can watch him perform Anne!"

"Perform?"

"All his little tricks of obedience."

He was writing. Laboriously, by hand. They stood on each side of the perfumed and primped boy in blonde ringlets and a neat black dress and tights that sat copying.

They read:

"Bill stood facing the boy. "Turn around." He ordered. The boy turned his eighteen year-old body towards the soldier. He came behind him and gently slid his thin white panties down. He felt his bottom cheeks gently. Then in went his drill… The boy gasped with pleasure…"

They watched as he wrote.

"That's enough!" Said Penelope.

"Make us tea."

He at-once obeyed.

He returned presently and served the young ladies.

"Kneel."

At her side.

"I shall ask Steven around." She said. She phoned.

He appeared soon. A man of twenty. Sporty of appearance.

"Open your mouth."

Steven was terribly turned on by the sight of the feminised slave. Obediently, he opened.

Steven stood in front of him. He gently, ever so gently took him in his mouth. He knew men loved to be gently teased.

"I bet he can make you cum, Steven."

"Bet you he can't!"

It was a contest.

It was so interesting to use every known skill in stroking, tonguing and teasing. Steven held firm, but it was remorseless. No pause. Endlessly teasingly, lickingly... He felt his balance slip mentally, and a hot... wet...

X

"Well Penelope?" Said Lady Fitzallan, "How's the new servant?"

"Fine, mother."

"Make sure you re-educate as well as dominate."

Penelope knew this. He must know where he fitted in the world-order. This meant he must be taught, told. His story told in many ways to him.

Penelope and her mother went to watch him.

He was placed in a chair, with his hands securely tied to the arms. The headphones repeated the stories. They listened as a new story began…

"Emma and Kate were astonished! So this was what Robert used to read!

It was a story with very strange content. They decided to catch him out. Later that day, while they were watching TV.

"I found out something strange!" Said Emma.

"What?" Said Kate.

"Some boys…"

"What?"

"Like to wear dresses."

"Really?"

"Like Sissies."

"Yes. Oh how cute!"

Robert flamed red.

"I'd love to see one!"

"Would you?"

"Someone pretty."

Robert got up and went upstairs. On his bed he saw something. Shocked… he flustered. They were green and very pretty.

The girls crept upstairs.

"Go on Robert, put them on!"

"I…"

They smiled. "Robert, we know. Do you want us to tell Mum?"

"No."

"Or Dad?"

"No."

Then put them on."

He obeyed nervously.

"Now Robert, you will be our slave. This is our little secret."

They laughed and left him to experience fear and bliss…"

"Re-educated to serve!"
"Quite"
"Indoctrinated."
Lady Fitzallan born to rule. Admired her daughter.

XI

"Yes."

"Please, No."

"Yes. Suck."

"No, please."

She slapped his face. Then pulled his hair-back and forced his mouth open. He came behind him laughing.

"Little slut, eh?"

"Take his arms Graham." She said.

Arms pulled back and tied, he was less resistant.

"He thinks it's too big." She said.

"You hold him while I…"

She took his position behind his bound arms.

"Relax, love." She soothed. "It's good."

Very powerful, Graham unzipped. "Come on." He said. At first he was gentle, but it was so huge.

He began to ram. "Suck bitch, slut. Come on slut! Use your tongue!"

"Ahh…"

"That's better!"

"Shh darling. Love your new role." Soothed Penelope.

"You dirty little slut!" He said.

"Now, lay him on his back."

On his back, arms tied, he stood over…

"Open wide!"

Like a dentist with his drill!

"Deep!"

"Come on love. He's your Master!"

"Do you like lollipops?" He panted.

The huge thing forced its way. "What a fucking sexy little bitch-whore slut you are!"

"This is your mission in life. Your true self darling." She stroked his legs.

He came and went.

Later she dressed him. "My pretty doll," she said.

She daubed big round spots of blush on his cheeks to accentuate the toy-doll look and black eyeliner.

"Later, I'll tie you to the bed." She said.

"Slave…"

64

XII

"Write!"

…Dear Tom,

I dream about you all the time, your lovely legs and those baggy jeans, which look so daring and sexy. Please let me come to your place and wear my sexiest clothes for you.

I want to stroke your legs, so softly and teasingly, to turn you on so your pole stands straight and gently ease it into my mouth."

"That will do, now add another…"

He told me to sit next to him. I obeyed.

"Now… Tell me." He said. "What do you think about?"

"Sex." I said.

"Tell me."

"I think about men."

"What about them?"

"Their big cocks."

"What do you think about them?"

"About touching them"

He laughed. "I'll show you one!"

He unzipped his jeans.

"Touch it."

I obeyed. It was hot and strong.

"Kiss it."

I obeyed.

"Lick."

I licked and sucked.

"Oh!" He gasped meaningfully. Then he got rough…

"You bitch!"

"Bitch-slut, lie flat on your back. Let me see your stockings."

I lay flat.

He pulled up my skirt and then knelt on me, straddling me, forcing his big dick into my mouth.

"Take it you whore." He obviously liked girls! I sucked as he thrust.

"You dirty little slut!" He complimented. He ran his hand under my panties, and found my chastity belt.

He rubbed.

I felt nothing. This increased my frustration to breaking point. He laughed.

"Suffer bitch!" He said and came in great oozes over my face…

"Pretty crude." She said.
"I'm sorry."
She laughed and ruffled my hair.
"My little slave…"

XIII

"I caught my brother; James, when he was sixteen, he was a slim and gorgeous young man, Penelope, wearing an old skirt."

"Oh." Said Penelope.

"He was just sixteen and it was an old one of mums. He was horrendously embarrassed; I asked him if he was a pervert. He was so frightened. I told him he'd need a Doctor, help, a psychiatrist. Dad must know. He was terrified."

"Really?"

"So I took my chance. I knew he was malleable. I told him I would tell Mum and Dad unless…"

"…Yes?"

"Well, Dad's ex-army and very big and powerful. A proper man." She laughed.

"Oh!" Said Penelope.

"So I bought him a pair of panties. Yellow, creamy. I made him kiss and stroke them and say 'I love my panties. I love them.' But I wouldn't let him near them 'till he'd got a pair of his own. I went with him to a shop in town and stood at the side, examining bras, while he had to ask for a pair in pink, just like the yellow ones…

…He nearly died of shame, but he did it. So next day, I made him buy some in green and explicitly say 'They are for my size?' The young assistant burst out laughing…

…When he had five pairs, I told him he must get a bra too. He wanted to resist, but I wasn't having any of it. So he bought a 34A, matching his panties, in white.

So we tried them on his lovely hairless soft body. I fastened it so slowly and pulled up the panties thinking: 'You are going to be such a slave!'

He had to write out: I love my bra. I love my panties, dozens of times and I got him to speak it into a tape and I gave the tape to my friend, Liz, who passed it around her friends.

Then we moved onto tights. He had to spend all his pocket money on tights of different shades and a slip. One Saturday when Mum and Dad were on holiday, Jennifer, my sister came to stay. She was twenty and I told her about my secret. She was shocked, but excited. We hooked out an old dress, but still pretty, and we cornered him.

He wanted to resist but the image of Dad settled it.

Jennifer went shopping. She said she 'wanted to meet her new sister' when she got back.

I made him obey. Panties and bra, tights, slip, the dress, shoes and then I made up his face with his lovely doe, soulful eyes.

"What are you going to do when you leave school?" She went on.

"College, I suppose."

"What are you going to study?"

"Art and design, I guess."

She laughed. "Very macho! Why don't you do fashion and beauty?"

I blushed.

Some weeks later I did start my Art and Design course. But Kate also did a course in hairdressing and body massage, part-time. So I used to see her around the college. I had a mate called Tony who was in his third year and nearly nineteen.

He used to like to look at my art portfolio and we knocked around together. He was into sixties screen-goddesses and stuff, but was always fun to be with and had a crowd of mates who he sang with in a sort of rock band.

"Why don't you come and sing along with us?" He said. But I was too shy at first. Kate noticed his interest in me and introduced herself, one lunchtime, while we sat in the college grounds.

"So… You're Tony. I've heard about you."

"And who are you?"

"I'm Kate."

"She's my sister." I said.

"So, you're in a rock band?" Said Kate.

"Sure, I play a bit."

"What?"

"Bass."

"Ooh!" Said Katie, "Very sexy."

Tony grinned.

"I've been trying to persuade your kid brother to come and join us."

"Oh, he's too shy."

I blushed. "Besides, he can't play anything."

"We like people to come along and sing."

"Really?"

"It's the group experience."

"Oh." Said Kate. "He's a good dancer."

"I'm not!" I said.

"I'll teach you."

"But…"

"But nothing. Perhaps you could dance to the songs onstage."

I blushed furiously: 'Me' as a dancer onstage?!?

"Great idea, we'll get a troupe of dancers to accompany the songs!" Said Tony.

I knew this mood. Kate was determined. She was going to get me to dance to Tony's songs come what may.

"We're giving a gig on the eighteenth, can you come and learn them a good week before?"

"Sure! We'll both come."

"Fantastic!" Said Tony.

And so it was! She borrowed his discs and listened to the songs then we began to work out routines together.

XV

"I began slowly – the day of our wedding."

"Tell me." Said Penelope.

"It was why I married him. I wanted someone to lead down the hill, all the way. Lower and lower."

"Yes."

"The reception was over. He had married me. Our honeymoon chalet was in view."

"'Now you are mine at last' he said with male inverted logic."

"Yes." Said Penelope.

"It's quite harmless. But you sleep soundly and he did. He woke up to find…"

"Yes?"

"I was still quite unconsummated of course."

"Quite."

"…To find a device."

"A device?"

"Attached to his…"

"…His?"

"So he could never…"

"…Never…"

"Molest me. He was astounded. Pleaded. Shouted. Begged. Fell on his knees. 'Where is the key?' I challenged him to ask someone to help him. Explain! 'My wife has locked me into a chastity cage!'"

Laughter!

"We returned from honeymoon, the happy couple!"

"We got used to the fact of my unlimited power. I told him 'release' would follow when…

After some weeks he was growing restless, so we went further."

"Further?"

"It is well known that eunuchs can only gain pleasure from certain pain."

"Yes."

"We began."

"And…?"

"I enjoyed teasing his frustration."

"Yes."

"And we had dinner parties where he served. Served food at first as an obvious slave and later…"

"Later?"

"Other services."

"To…?"

"…To women, and men."

"Ah…"

"And dressed appropriately."

"Dressed?"

"In feminine costumes."

"Ahh, yes."

"There are things to consider Penelope. They must taste the depths. Of total submission… Deeper and deeper."

"Yes."

They sipped iced tea very sedately.

XVI

"Please no."

"Yes."

"Please."

She turned away.

"It's settled. He will be here in ten minutes."

"Please."

"Shut up." Said Penelope. "Go and put on your delicious soft spangled jeans and little boots. I want you looking androgynous."

Meekly, he came back.

"Just a tiny hint of lipstick. You look delicious." His face hung down.

"Darling relax, I'm only loaning you." The doorbell rang.

"Ah, James!"

"Penelope!"

"Here he is."

"Hi there." He said, conscious of suave and soothing manner he loved to exude. It said 'I Charm…'

Penelope watched them shake hands. She knew what was in store. James was a noted seducer. He had trails of women after him.

She wanted him to use his full panoply on her slave.

"Remember," she hissed, "Your job is to please."

He was scared.

When men like James touched you, you quivered and submitted. They filled you with hopeless longings. They drove to one of James' luxury apartments in London.

"Hi Sophie!" He said to a kind of maid. "This is my friend."

"Hi!" Said Sophie then and left.

"Sophie cleans for me. She's just going."

"Goodnight Mr James!" The door closed.

"Well, we're alone."

"Yes."

"Are you scared?"

He nodded.

"Don't be. I won't hurt you. I think you're very beautiful. Very attractive, I want to make you feel like a million guineas. I am going to gently melt your resistance with delicate soothing caresses. I want you to know your beauty, darling. To feel how precious you are. How sublime. Let me stroke your hand and tease away your fear."

Gently, he held his hand.

"Shhh… Let me stroke you into oblivion…

"...That's better. Now give me your other hand. Good sweetheart. Let me gently caress your wrists."

"Good."

"Later sweetheart, I am going to...

...But now, let me kiss you."

"That's right. Surrender."

"Oh,"

"Shhh."

"Relax." He said.

"It's not true that I break hearts." Said James. "I break minds. I break resistance."

"Oh."

"Now, give yourself."

Remorselessly, James grew. Soon he was invading the spangled jeans, which lay discarded.

"Moan for me." Said James.

James loved the sense of another surrender, yet another. He loved that feeling of totally expert fucking, which left women desperate for a repeat.

...And he loved the feeling of this boy being one of his conquered girls.

XVII

Penelope watched him squirm.

"So you want to go back to him?"

He nodded ashamed.

"For the joy of being so expertly fucked, so delicately seduced and invaded."

He hung his head.

"To become his slave. To do anything for the pleasure of touching his lovely dick, caressing it and licking."

He stared at the ground.

"You've become a quivering mass of weak girl. Look at you, in sexy stockings and short skirt." She laughed.

"He'll take you and use you like a rag then cast you amid his discards. One of his anxious slaves, he'll pass you to his friends to serve like a helpless, hopeless trollop."

He gasped.

"Go on, beg for it. Beg for his mighty dick in you, spearing and controlling and entering."

"I want you to long for it, to be desperate."

"Go on. Beg!"

"Beg to be fucked!"

"Oh, please!" He gasped. "I need it!"

She laughed. She telephoned.

He heard his master's voice. He laughed. "He is coming over." She said. "To fix you in dependence."

XVIII

"Amazing Penny."

"I'm glad you like it Karen."

"Entrancing. You know, when I was sixteen, I made my brother dress up once."

"Really?"

"He was watching me get dressed for the school prom."

"Oh!"

"And he must have seen me naked."

"Oh."

"So, like Diana, the Goddess, I decided to punish him."

"Really?"

"I said: 'So you like panties do you?'"

"'No' He said."

"'I don't believe you. Put these on, or I'll tell Dad you were spying on me.'"

"'They're tight…'"

"'Good. Now a bra.'"

"'No, please.'"

"'Yes. Now tights'"

"'Please.'"

"'Go on, you'll love it.'"

"'Please no.'"

"'Shut up, or I'll tell.'"

"'Sorry.'

"'Now, a nice little skirt and top'"

"'No, please.'"

"'Do you feel guilty?'"

"'Yes.'"

"'Let's do your face.'"

"'No please.'"

"'And hair.'"

"'No, please!'"

"'Yes!' Then I took photos"

"Honestly?"

"Yes."

He lay at Penelope's feet stroking her.

"Isn't he cute?"

"Yes."

"He's very dreamy."

"He's dreaming of James and his big cock."

They giggled.

"Aren't you darling?"

She petted him.

"You see, men are all the same. They are weak and helpless. We women have the task of subduing them. Either by force, by teasing delight and enchantment or both."

They looked at him in his very short skirt, extremely pretty.

He was their slave.

Academy Incorporated
- turning fantasy into reality -

Does a reform school where adult boys, girls and special girls relive or rewrite their schooldays appeal? Or maid training for work with us at Muir Academy or as historical role-play with real spanking and bondage, or elsewhere? Or would you like to be a Master, Mistress, slave, human pony or puppy in that village? Or do you want mail-order books, magazines, implements, audio and video tapes, adult-size school or maid uniform?

We help one and all to do such things, men and women, 18 to 80s, married, couple or single; cross-dressers, transsexuals, heterosexuals, bisexuals, homosexuals, Dominants, switches, submissives, the short, tall, fat or thin, beginner or those who've done it all, able- bodied or otherwise, any race or religion. Discreetly too, and in safety, since 1987.

For free info.

contact:

PO Box 135, Hereford, HR2 7WL, UK

www.tawse.com, email: guy@tawse.com

or ring 01432 343100